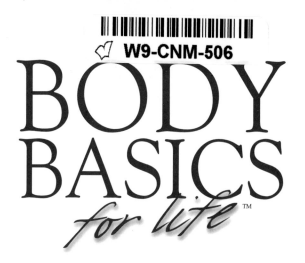

BODY BASICS
for life™

Simple steps to a healthy,
pain-free you!

Here's what people are saying about
BODY BASICS *for life*

"Thank you for writing an intelligent, practical outline of lifestyle activities which are easy to adopt. This is invaluable advice for parents and others providing children's education."

"A great lifestyle reference for physician office practice – for waiting room reading."

ELEANOR HOWIE PhC.
PHARMACEUTICAL CHEMIST & RECEIVER OF CARE

"This book explains, in personable and easy-to-understand terminology, a common-sense approach to a healthy lifestyle and a fitter you."

DAVID WILLIAMS. M.D.

"A cost-effective way to radically change the focus of health care in our country — from lengthy expensive treatment of disease to inexpensive prevention of disease."

DIANNE ZAKARIA. M.Sc.P.T., MCPA

"If more of these good habits were practised earlier in life, it would help reduce musculoskeletal problems present in our Olympic and professional athletes and thus improve their performance."

KAREN ORLANDO B.Sc.P.T.. B.Sc.H.K.
CONSULTANT TO THE TORONTO RAPTORS AND CANADA'S NATIONAL ROWING TEAM

"**Body Basics** *for life* is an excellent resource for people taking an active role in adopting a healthy lifestyle."

SHARON SWITZER-McINTYRE B.P.E.. B.Sc.P.T., M.ED.
ASSISTANT PROFESSOR. UNIVERSITY OF TORONTO

"This guide to physical well being is logical, readable and beautifully illustrated. However, what sets it apart from other health guides is the author's ability to look at health and postural issues from both sides of the fence. She has treated and helped resolve the problems of hundreds of patients of all ages through her work as a practising physiotherapist. She has also had the experience of chronic discomfort and has learnt the hard way that there is no quick fix but rather daily attention to posture, flexibility and muscle strength can dramatically reduce discomfort and improve quality of life."

ERIC LENCZNER M.D.. FRCS(C)
ORTHOPAEDIC SURGEON
CONSULTANT TO THE MONTREAL CANADIENS AND MONTREAL ALOUETTES

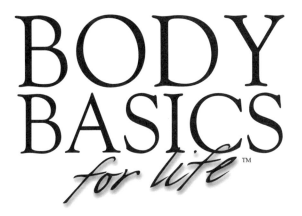

BODY BASICS *for life*™

Simple steps to a healthy,
pain-free you!

For Your Health!

Karen Webb

Karen Webb
B.P.T., MCPA

Birchcliff Publishing Inc.
Stratford, Ontario, Canada

Body Basics for life is a trademark of Birchcliff Publishing Inc.

Canadian Cataloguing in Publication Data.

Webb, Karen, 1953–
 Body Basics for life: simple steps to a healthy, pain free you!

Includes bibliographical references.
ISBN 0-9682571-0-0

1. Posture.   2. Physical fitness.   I. Title.
RA781.5.W42 1997   613.7'8   C97-900865-4

Inside Design by Janet Keen.
Photography by Michael McClintock.
Editing by Layne Verbeek.
Cover Design by Heidi Holdsworth.
Cover & Author Photo by Elisabeth Feryn.
Chair Prop on Cover: property of the Stratford Festival
Printed in Canada by The Beacon Herald Fine Printing Division, Stratford, Ontario.

All inquiries should be addressed to:
Birchcliff Publishing Inc.
Suite 126, 59 Albert Street
Stratford, Ontario
N5A 3K2
(519) 273-3334
E-mail: birchclf@orc.ca

Quantity discounts are available on bulk purchases of this book. For information contact Birchcliff Publishing Inc. at the above address or call us at (519) 273-3334 or toll free at 1-888-472-9121. A mail-order form is located in the back of the book.

To each and every one of us:
May we fill our minds with knowledge
and free our bodies from pain!

ACKNOWLEDGEMENTS

Inside Design by Janet Keen
Photography by Michael McClintock
Editing by Layne Verbeek
Cover Design by Heidi Holdsworth
Cover & Author Photograph by Elisabeth Feryn
Cover chair prop courtesy of the Stratford Festival

Paul Webb, my partner in life, is the driving force behind this project and I mean that literally — our quiet talk time is often during our long journeys to and from the lake, while our daughters sleep. **Body Basics for life** was born somewhere along a winding country road.

Dianne Zakaria is a physiotherapist who helped me when I had problems with my neck and back and I still see her regularly at the YMCA. Dianne has been a great resource, both in helping me with my physical health as well as supporting me on this project. Dianne is returning to university for a doctorate program.

Erin Carson is a kinesiology student who I met while exercising at the YMCA. Erin is living proof that the information in **Body Basics for life** works! She is energetic, enthusiastic and full of ideas. I thank Erin for her support.

Dean Robinson, a Stratford author, has always been available to answer my questions and provide sound advice. More interestingly, Dean was one of my first patients when I graduated as a physiotherapist.

My sincere thanks go to the following people who have been there for me when I needed support and encouragement: Nancy Algie, David Carter, Nancy Coldham, Linda Hatton, Signe Holstein, Jane Kirkpatrick, Dianne Millette, Janet and Greta Podleski (authors of Looneyspoons™), Ellen Young, and all the helpful staff at the Stratford Public Library.

CONTENTS

MY STORY

Your body is important to you. Yet the wear and tear of everyday living on your body is magnified by the onslaught of computers, video games and other modern forms of automation. Prolonged sitting and body neglect take their toll, as we see aches and strains showing up earlier in life. Do you want to avoid pain? Do you want your body to last? How about your child's body? Then this book is for you!

It's subtitled *Simple steps to a healthy, pain-free you!* because that's what I promise to teach you. The simple tasks in this book will make it easy for you and your loved ones to understand the causes of unnecessary body pain and how to avoid them.

We place tremendous physical stress on ourselves everyday: with prolonged sitting at desks and computer terminals, with improper warm-up for sports, with repetitive activities, and even with poor standing, resting postures and sleeping habits. The long-term effects develop innocently, are often overlooked, but then become chronic. Now is the time to become better informed, develop a healthy physical body, and help the generations that follow in your footsteps.

I should know. As a physiotherapist with more than twenty years' experience, and the proud mother of two beautiful children, I found no time for myself. After years of ignoring the pain in my neck and back, I finally sought help from a professional associate. I could have avoided excruciating pain and suffering had I practised the same healthy physical habits I promote as a physiotherapist.

An old Yiddish proverb says, "Trouble brings experience and experience brings wisdom." I've had the trouble and learned the hard way with my own experiences. I've shared my hard-won wisdom with both my husband and our kids. Now, I want to share my new lifestyle habits with you.

"From the errors of others, a wise man corrects his own."

PUBLIUS SYRUS,
MORAL SAYINGS

Eight out of ten people experience back pain. In most cases of physical complaints, the pain could have been avoided if the person had the right information or know-how. The basic lessons in this book will help you solve many postural complaints as well as help you prevent health problems.

As you will see, I've provided lots of practical information with photographs. I cover a variety of health topics, which include: good sitting and standing postures; survival exercises for the neck and back; and abdominal crunches. I have also included tips for carrying purses, briefcases and backpacks.

I will also show you how to avoid muscular problems associated with repetitive activities such as computer keyboarding and piano playing. Along the way, I discuss the young athlete and his or her growth spurts, issues related to fat and lean bodies, user-friendly desk work, and a number of aerobic and other exercise programs.

You will also find helpful checklists for classrooms, the gym and the workplace at the end of this book. Finally, I have an all-inclusive checklist which is also available in a condensed version as a poster.

No one should suffer unnecessary pain and discomfort. These healthy habits and simple exercises will start you and your family on the way to a happy and pain-free life.

Karen Webb

BENDING

Your spine consists of your neck, mid-back, low back, sacrum (triangular bone below your low back) and tail bone. Jelly doughnut-like discs separate the bones in your neck, mid-back and low back allowing for movement. The neck has a tremendous amount of rotation, allowing you to safely look over your shoulder when driving a car or riding a bike. Rotation in your lower back is small and this is why we hear about lower back twisting type injuries.

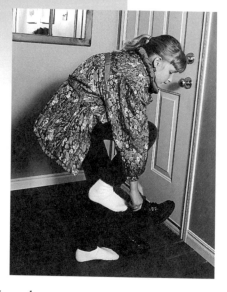

One big mistake we tend to make is that we do not keep our necks and lower backs mobile. We tend to move our spine in one direction repeatedly but seldom in the opposite direction. The most common excess movement we do in our lower back is forward bending, such as tying a shoe or sitting in a chair. The most common excess movements in our neck are forward bending combined with a poking of our heads forward. As a physiotherapist I saw many people with conditions developing from excess movement that they could have prevented. The movements we must also do regularly are backward bending of our lower backs and backward bending of our necks.

We bend forward too often during the day.

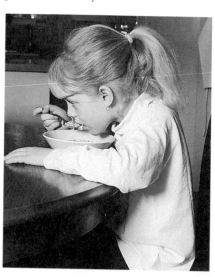

10

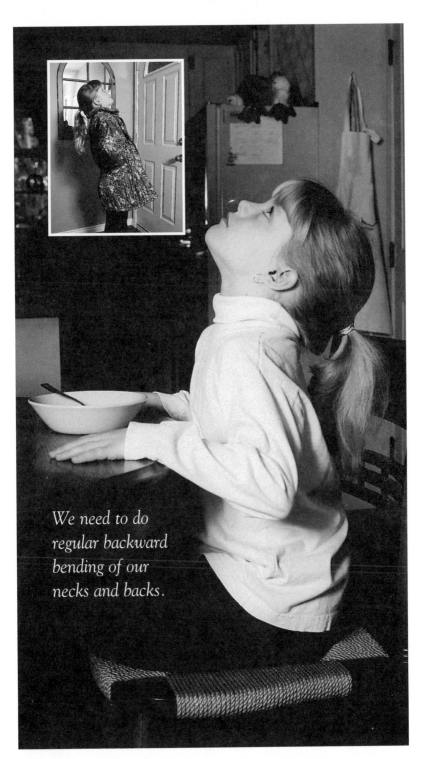

We need to do regular backward bending of our necks and backs.

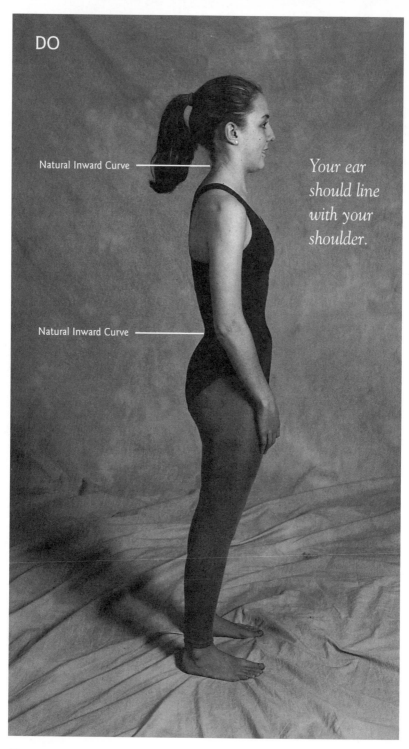

DO

Natural Inward Curve ————

Natural Inward Curve ————

Your ear should line with your shoulder.

POSTURES FOR LIFE

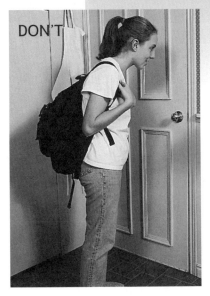

DON'T

Your neck has a natural inward curve, or hollow just above your shoulders. When standing upright your ears should line with your shoulders. As a result of not paying attention or not knowing, people carry their heads in front of their bodies with their chins poking forward.

Your lower back also has a natural inward curve, or hollow. This hollow is lost when your lower back is rounded from a poor sitting posture or when you are bent forward.

Robin McKenzie, an internationally respected physiotherapist from New Zealand, is recognized as an expert in neck and back pain. He believes poor posture, in the long term, can be just as harmful as an injury. He also believes most deformities in the elderly are the visible effects of long-standing poor habits and are, most importantly, preventable. I for one, agree with Robin McKenzie's statement in his book *Treat Your Own Back*, "...spinal pain of a postural origin would not occur if basic education were given to individuals at an early age."

Deformities in the elderly can be seen as the visible side-effects of poor posture started in the young.

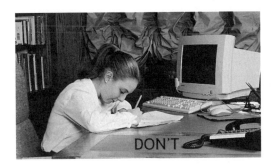

DON'T

SITTING

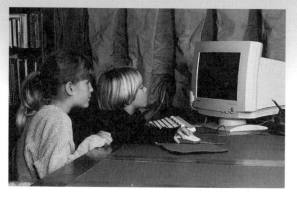

Today, children sit even longer with TV, video games and computers.

Watch how you sit. Muscles that support your lower back get tired. With muscle fatigue, the inward curve, or hollow in your lower back, is lost and you slouch. Muscles that support your head and neck also tire and the inward curve in your neck is lost and your head and neck poke forward. Once the slouched posture of your lower back takes over, it is next to impossible to maintain good posture of your head and neck. In the past, poor head and neck posture developed around the mid-teens when the length of time sitting increased with schoolwork and homework. Today children sit for longer hours in front of the television, video games and computers, and risk developing a poor posture at an *even earlier* age.

Practise. Learn to feel the difference between good and bad posture.

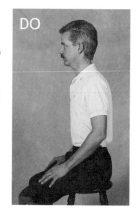

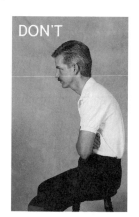

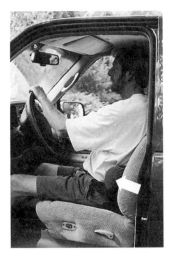

Avoid sitting without a backrest for long periods of time. A slouching posture will slowly take over no matter how hard you try to avoid it. Did you know that your back muscles may get more of a workout when you sit on the football bleachers than the players do on the field? Some chairs do provide good support to our lower back but most do not. We have to be prepared to add our own lower back support.

I take my low back roll everywhere. It can be used in any chair, sofa, car or theatre seat. You simply place the roll in the small of your back at your waistline. If you drive a lot, keep a roll in your car for extra support. Back rolls are available at most pharmacies and medical supply stores. Density of foam varies, so try each one out for comfort.

Another healthy habit for you and your family is to take breaks from long periods of sitting. Simple stretching exercises take barely a minute to perform. These exercises have grown close to my heart and are fondly referred to as 'survival exercises' (see pages 18 to 21). Robin McKenzie is credited for these exercises, and many more, all of which appear in his self-treatment books.

Simple stretching exercises take barely a minute to perform.

You'll see that most children move around a lot, even during activities that require sitting. Parents think their children are fidgety, but in reality, they are doing what their bodies are telling them to do. Who knows more about body basics, Mom and Dad or the children?

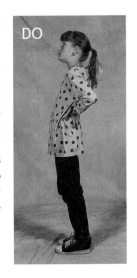

DO

USER-FRIENDLY DESK WORK

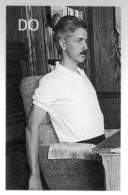

Every day, young and old sit at tables or desks reading, completing assignments, writing essays or working at their computers. While we sit and do these activities, we often position ourselves in harmful or bad postures. Some of us sit forward on the edge of our chair, hunched over with our heads buried in a book. Others cross their legs or twist one leg around the other like a pretzel. Some lean on one elbow creating a sideward curve in their spine. And, some have their arms held out, unsupported, while typing. All of these activities have the same result — we end up with sore necks, backs and shoulders, and sometimes a headache.

Save your back: interrupt keyboarding, relax, hang your arms at your sides and bend backwards a few times while sitting.

TELEPHONE

Poor telephone habits are common.

Always hold the receiver in your hand. Don't tuck it between your head and shoulder. Tucking the phone between your ear and shoulder may give you free hands today — but this will only give you a neck problem tomorrow. I suggest you buy a speaker phone or head set if you find you're using the phone a lot.

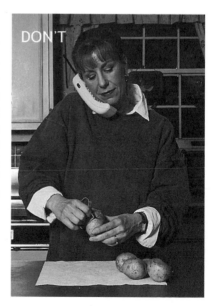

SEATING

- Support the inward curve in your lower back with a back roll or rolled up towel if your chair doesn't have adequate support
- Keep your feet flat on your foot rest or flat on the floor
- Make sure your seat supports you from your hips to your knees
- Make sure your knees fit comfortably under your desk

KEYBOARDING

- Keep your arms at the sides of your body
- Keep your elbows bent at 90°
- Hold your forearms and wrists parallel to the floor (as seen in the photo below)

SCREEN

- Sit about one arm's length back from the screen
- Position your monitor so the top line of print is level with your eyes
- Keep your head and neck upright

Healthy Hints

Be computer wise:

- Stretch arms, hands, neck and back every sixty minutes or even sooner if you feel a strain

- Walk around every once in awhile

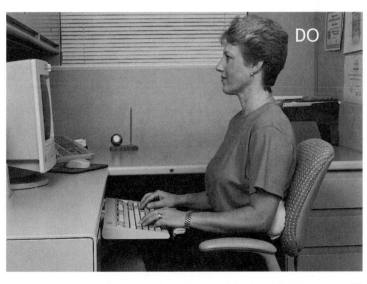

DO

SURVIVAL EXERCISES

'SLOPPY' PUSH-UP

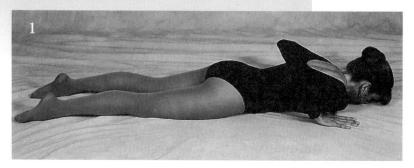

1. Lie face down and place your hands under your shoulders

2. Straighten your elbows and allow your back to sag.
   Hold this for two counts

Repeat this exercise five to 10 times

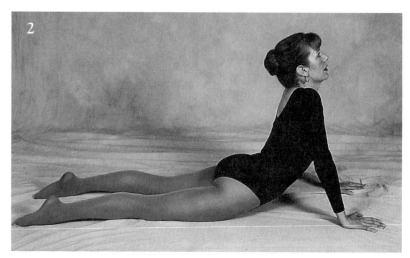

Healthy Hints

Do 'sloppy' push-ups:

• As part of your morning routine

• As part of your night routine

• Before and after every abdominal muscle workout

BACK BEND

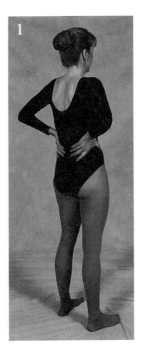

1. While standing, place your hands in the small of your back, with your fingers pointing inwards

2. Bend backwards at your waist keeping your knees straight. Hold this for two counts

Repeat this exercise five times

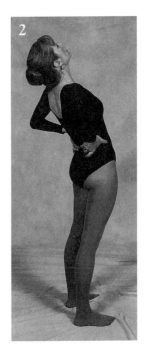

Healthy Hints

Do back bends:

• Prior to and during repeated lifting

• While sitting for long periods of time

• Following every strenuous workout

• When you feel minor strains developing in your back

CHIN TUCK

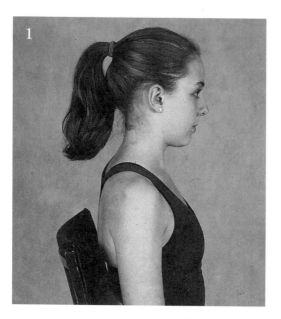

1. Sit with good back posture. Look straight ahead and relax

2. Move your head straight back with your eyes looking forward. Imagine you have a plate of peas on top of your head that you don't want to spill. Hold this for two counts

Repeat this exercise five times

Healthy Hints

Do chin tucks:

- As part of your morning routine

- As part of your night routine

- While doing desk work for long periods of time

- After every strenuous workout

- After every abdominal muscle workout that strains your neck

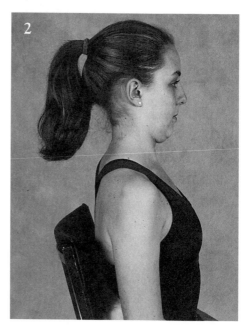

BACKWARD NECK BEND

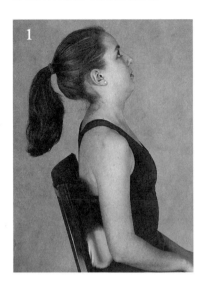

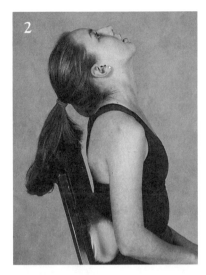

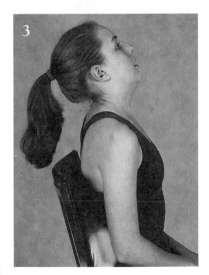

1. While holding your 'chin tuck', tilt your head backwards

2. Let go of your chin tuck to allow you to move your head back as far as comfortably possible.
   Hold this for two counts

3. As you bring your head up, regain your chin tuck and then return to an upright position

Repeat this exercise five times

Healthy Hints

Do backward neck bends:

- While doing desk work for long periods of time

- After every abdominal muscle workout that strains your neck

- After sleeping on your stomach

DO

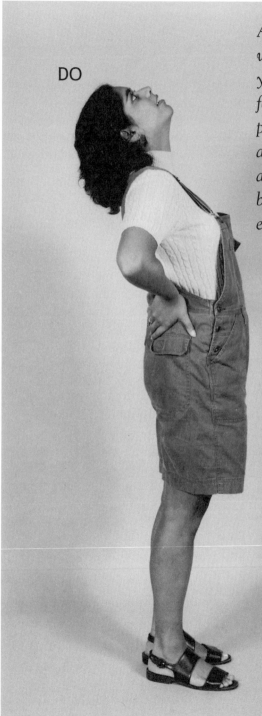

Always interrupt work that requires you to stand bent forward. This is a position of strain and should be avoided. Do five back bends whenever possible.

STANDING

When standing for a long time, the muscles that support your body get tired and lazy. Your natural low-back hollow becomes excessive. This can result in a 'sway back' over time. Young teenagers, particularly if they're tall, can feel awkward amongst their peers. As a result they often slouch in an attempt to go unnoticed and develop poor posture habits. Remind them to stand upright, just like the army commands from old movies: "Stand Tall, Chest Up and Stomach In!"

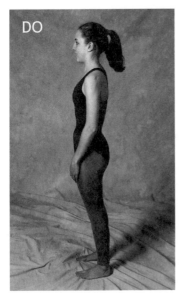

We all stand bent over for many activities: children at craft tables, teenagers over microscopes, and parents at the kitchen counter. Whenever you do things that have you bent forward for long periods of time, give your back a regular stretch break and do five back bends as demonstrated on the opposite page.

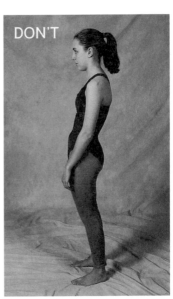

Practise good posture: Stand Tall, Chest Up, Stomach In!

RESTING

MATTRESS

The comfort and support given by a mattress is affected by the base it is placed on. When buying a mattress it is best to place it on a box spring of similar quality. If you will be placing it on a solid base, try it out before you buy it by placing it on the floor to see how it will feel. Avoid mattresses that sag or are too hard.

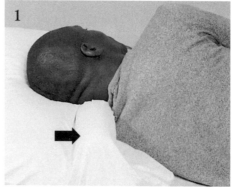

PILLOWS

Babies start off in cribs with no pillows. Somewhere along the way, many of us inherit more than one, or often an over-stuffed pillow. Sleeping with a crook in your neck will likely result in neck complaints early in life. Remember, one pillow is enough! Since your pillow should support your head and neck, the pillow needs to fill the hollow between your head and shoulders. Feather or foam chip pillows work well since you can adjust their shape to support your neck.

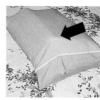

NECK ROLL INSIDE PILLOW

Neck rolls provide support to those who have difficulty getting adequate support from a pillow. The roll is placed inside the pillow case (as demonstrated in the photograph to the right). I take my neck roll on all overnight trips (it fits easily into a small space). I prefer to take my bed pillow, but this is not always possible.

Healthy Hints

1. Use one pillow to sleep or try a neck roll inside your pillow case if you need more support

2. Do five chin tucks when you wake up

3. Do five 'sloppy' push-ups when you wake up

4. If you have slept on your stomach, do five backward neck bends and turn your head to each side as if to look over your shoulders. Repeat five times

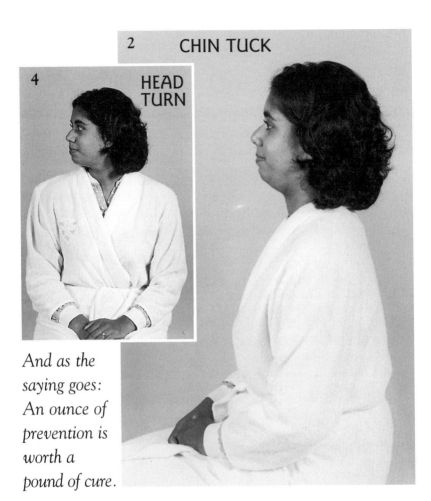

2   CHIN TUCK

4   HEAD TURN

And as the saying goes: An ounce of prevention is worth a pound of cure.

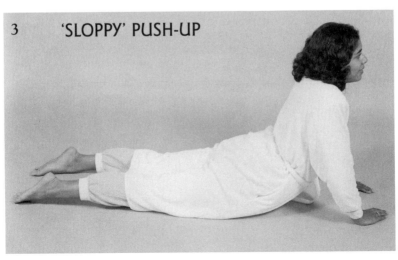

3   'SLOPPY' PUSH-UP

RELAXING

Think of what you do after a full day of golf, soccer or skiing. After any vigorous activity you probably relax. I love to ski and I know that feeling of accomplishment and exhaustion after I've spent a full day on the slopes. I, like most of us, like to relax in a big cozy chair by the fireplace sipping a hot drink. So, who thinks about their sitting posture? Over the years I have had friends develop back pain. Most of them attribute their pain to skiing, even though their pain did not begin until *after* they slouched in a big chair for an hour or two. They have now begun rolling up their ski jackets and using them as back rolls. I have also shown them how to do back bends and chin tucks after skiing. And don't forget, when you are drinking, to make sure you bring your drink to your mouth rather than poking your head forward to your cup.

Relaxing after vigorous activity can set you up for pain.

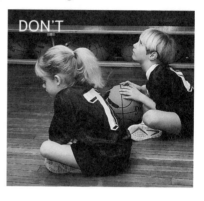

DON'T

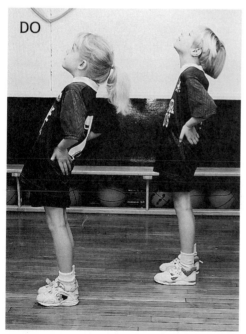

DO

Healthy Hints

- Perform five back bends and five chin tucks after every vigorous activity

- Pay attention to your posture when relaxing after a workout. If you're sitting, maintain your natural inward curves in your neck and back

- Use a low-back roll

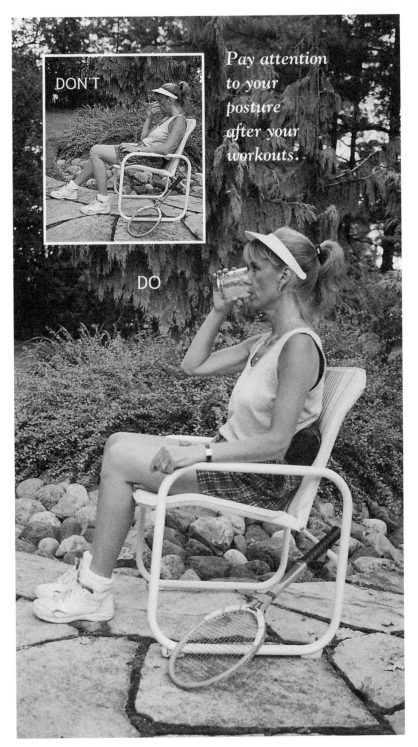

DON'T

Pay attention to your posture after your workouts.

DO

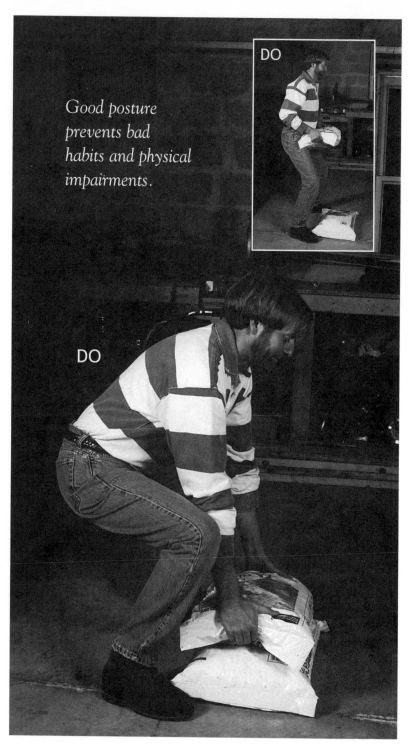

Good posture prevents bad habits and physical impairments.

DO

DO

LIFTING

As young children we have the right idea. Watch your children pick up a toy or a crayon from the floor. Children bend both knees and crouch to pick up the object, whether it is large or small, heavy or light. But, as children grow older, they develop the poor lifting and 'picking up' habits that are so often seen in adults. Bending forward from your waist to pick up an object, lifting an object that is far away from your body, or twisting while you lift, are all bad habits.

As children grow older, they develop the poor lifting and picking up habits so often seen in adults (as demonstrated in the photo to the right).

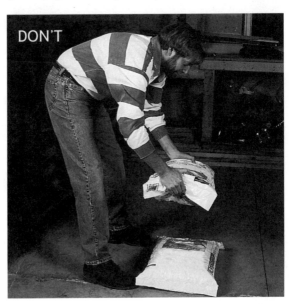

DON'T

Healthy Hints

- Do five back bends prior to lifting
- Stand close to the load and maintain a firm, wide stance
- Retain the hollow in your lower back
- Bend your knees and drop down to the load
- Hold the load close to your body
- Lift the load by straightening your knees
- When standing, shift your feet to avoid twisting your back

ABDOMINAL MUSCLES

LET'S CRUNCH TOGETHER

Abdominal muscles play an important role in many of our daily activities. Stronger abdominals assist us with good posture; hold our internal organs in place; enhance our appearance; and provide the strength necessary to improve our technique and performance during sports activities.

The traditional sit-up has been abandoned; it puts undue stress on the lower back. Abdominal crunches are now the exercises of choice, for these exercises minimize unnecessary movement and maximize muscle work.

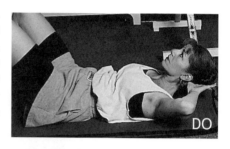

DO

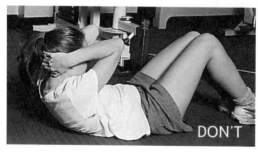

DON'T

- Support your head and lift it towards the ceiling so that your shoulder blades are just off the mat

- Do not pull your head or neck

Healthy Hints

- Support your head and neck with your finger tips

- Do not poke your chin or head forward if you must lift your head unsupported

- Perform five backward neck bends if you stress your neck

- Always start and end each abdominal workout with ten 'sloppy' push-ups

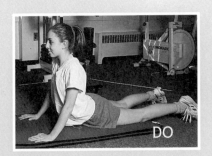

DO

Always do ten 'sloppy' push-ups before and after your abdominal workout.

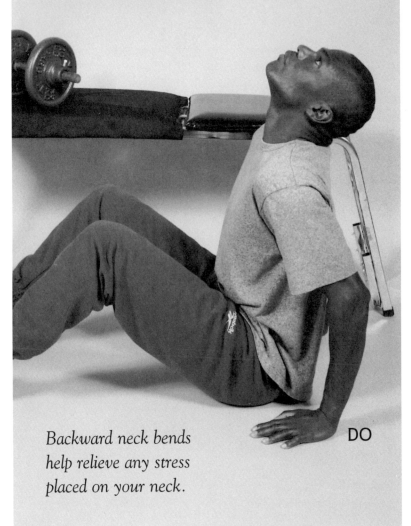

DO

Backward neck bends help relieve any stress placed on your neck.

BACKPACKS & PURSES

BACKPACKS

Backpacks are used from kindergarten to university. In the early days, the loads are light and Mom and Dad often carry the bags. By grade two though, the bags get heavier. They get filled with running shoes, lunches, library books and different toys for Show and Tell. By mid-highschool, bags can weigh up to 10 kilograms (22 pounds). Long-term, improper carrying of a heavy backpack can lead to poor posture, over-stretching of the soft tissue in your neck and back, and, ultimately, pain.

Use both shoulder straps of your backpack and stand tall.

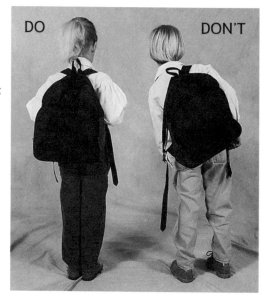

DO   DON'T

Healthy Hints

- Heavy backpacks should also have chest, waist or hip straps to help distribute the load more evenly across your body
- Backpacks for hiking and camping provide additional support through frames and special straps. Be sure to buy the right backpack for your body

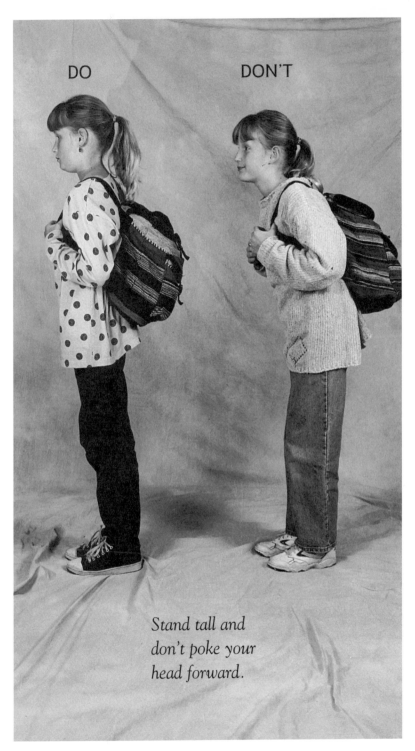

DO DON'T

Stand tall and don't poke your head forward.

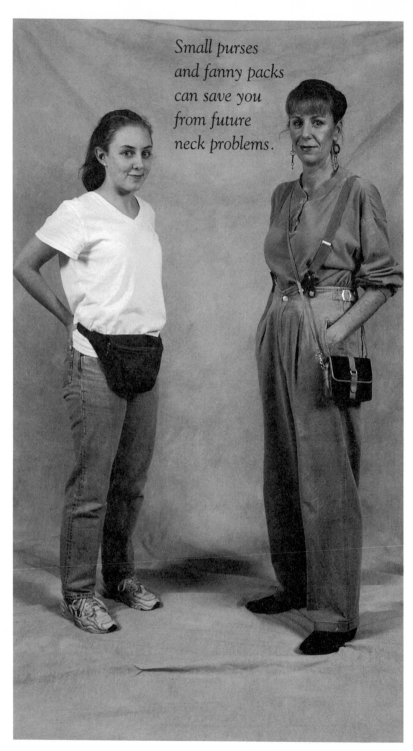

Small purses
and fanny packs
can save you
from future
neck problems.

PURSES

Most women carry a purse every day. Purses should be light and tucked under the arm. Shoulder straps should be worn across the body, rather than hung from one side. Carrying a heavy purse over your shoulder can lead to many physical complaints. More recently, I have been using a fanny pack or a small, light purse with the shoulder strap across my body (like the photo on the left). Both work well, but the biggest challenge is to reduce the load in your purse!

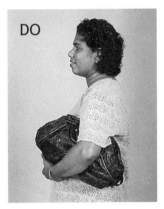

DO

Healthy Hints

- Use a small purse or fanny pack

- Carry your purse tucked under your arm and be sure to alternate the side you carry it on

- Keep your elbows slightly bent when carrying briefcases, suitcases and groceries

BRIEFCASES / CARRYBAGS

If you can't keep your elbow slightly bent when you carry a bag, then it is too heavy.

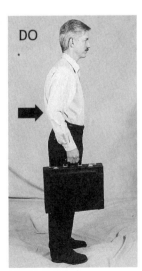

DO

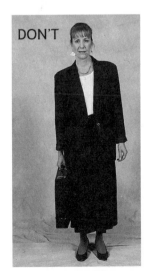

DON'T

TIRED MUSCLES

ARM YOURSELF AGAINST UPPER BODY ABUSE

We tend to take our arms and hands for granted. Yet our fingers, hands, wrists, elbows, and shoulders are all capable of a great deal of skill and grace. We can sew a button on a shirt, pick a crumb up off the table or turn a page in a book. We can cast a fishing line, play table tennis or turn a skipping rope. Our muscles work best when they are moving.

When you make your muscles work without movement, such as holding a sign above your head for several minutes, the blood supply to your muscles slows down. If you work at a keyboard for an hour, your muscles get tired and achy. Stress is placed on the nerves and blood vessels that run down the length of your arm. These get bent at your elbow just like a kink in a garden hose, interrupting the natural flow. Leaving these nerves bent for long periods of time can lead to painful problems.

The second harmful habit is when you perform repeated movements over long periods of time. This is how repetitive strain injuries develop. We don't realize what we are asking of these small muscles and joints when we intensively knit, type or play the piano.

Our arms are stronger in one direction of movement because of our regular and repeated daily activities. These muscles are the muscles that allow us to grip the handle of a suitcase or to hug someone. At the same time, the muscles that move our arms in the opposite direction are normally weaker since we use them less.

Healthy Hints

- Take a break from your activity and stretch every hour. The more intensive the activity, the more frequently you need to break

- If you feel a strain in your neck, arms or back: Stop and stretch! Mini breaks are sometimes needed

- Pace yourself with every project. Give your body parts a break when doing things like painting a fence, raking leaves or doing a puzzle

- Listen to your body. Pain is it's warning signal

- Remember to *stretch* your eyes and periodically look away from your television or computer

The muscles in your forearm that hold your wrist in position for typing are part of a weaker group of muscles. Not only do we keep our arms in one position for a long time, we also perform many repeated movements in our fingers as we type. These muscles are particularly at risk for injury.

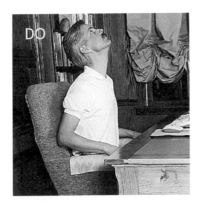

Take a break and stretch!

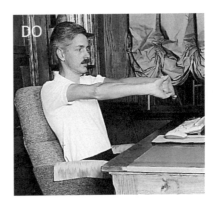

Performing repeated movements and holding our body in one position for a long time is body abuse.

EYES

Our eyes are also worked by muscles and these get tired just as other muscles in our body do.

- Avoid staring or over-stimulation, such as watching too much TV or staring at a computer screen

- Interrupt any activities requiring a lot of concentration and staring. Try focusing on different objects at different distances

- Practise blinking, for this also helps to combat the effects of staring by washing your eyes with your tears

FIT & FAT

FITNESS

A person's level of fitness does not stay constant. It changes in response to a number of factors, many of which we can either control or learn to control. Such factors include: good posture, proper exercise, adequate rest, proper diet and weight control. Fit people avoid excessive drinking. They also avoid smoking and using drugs. Getting proper medical care is also important. But, ignoring one area of your body's health can affect the good things you do for another part of your body. A diet aimed at weight loss and improved body composition must also include an exercise plan.

The wicked queen in Snow White demonstrates how many of us look at personal beauty and aging. However, physical attractiveness does not lie in one single body type because it is based on muscle development and fat distribution in proportion to the body frame. Physical attractiveness lies in each and every one of our body types. We must also accept our body's natural aging process and the changes that it will go through. However, we need to know what we *can* change in our bodies and *accept* what we cannot.

Good exercise will lead to improvements in our bodies, such as improved muscle tone and reduced body fat. Although most of us care about how we look and physical attractiveness can be improved with exercise, this should *not* be our reason for exercise. Exercise, relax and have fun, for when your body begins to feel good the rest will take care of itself.

"A healthy lifestyle should be part of a person's general culture, just like knowing Leonardo da Vinci painted the Mona Lisa."

DR. JACQUES GENEST JR., CLINICAL RESEARCH INSTITUTE OF MONTREAL

Healthy Hint

Exercise and proper diet help each of us reach and maintain our unique attractiveness

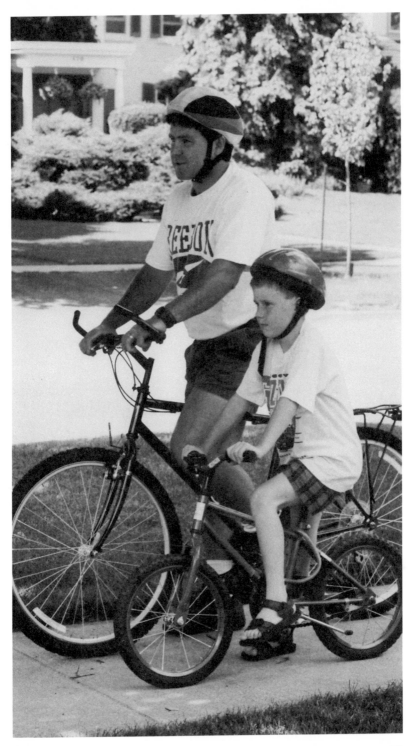

FIT AND FAT CHAT

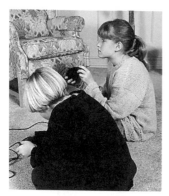

With television, video games, the home computer and now access to the Internet, our children have even more exciting things to do. As a result, our children sit for longer periods of time, often with poor posture. This puts them at risk for future physical problems. Recent studies found obesity increasing amongst pre-teen children and it links the rising amount of fat in a child's diet to the time spent in front of the TV. Even more startling, cardiologist Anthony Graham, advisor to the Heart and Stroke Foundation of Ontario, has identified fatty streaks in the blood vessels of children as young as three. Habits developed early in life are powerful! Just as we can teach our children good posture and lifting techniques, we should also teach our children proper eating habits and the importance of exercise.

Fast food restaurants are here to stay. Advertising is persuasive and even if you wish to stay away, children are insistent. Interestingly, when my children were about four years old, they told me they liked the toy more than the meal. Truth from the mouths of babes!

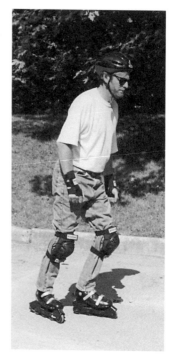

If you must visit your local fast food restaurant, here's a tip. Walk or roller blade to the restaurant. Go to the playground first, kick a soccer ball around or do some kind of physical activity. I suggest you try "Running and *then* Eating" rather than the more common approach of "Eating and

Healthy Hints

- "Run and Eat", rather than "Eat and Run"
- Walk or roller blade to the fast food restaurant instead of driving

Running." Calories continue to be burned after exercise and this exercise helps to control our appetites.

Numerous health risks are associated with excess body fat. Heart disease tops the list. In North America more people are overweight today than ten years ago – including children.

Basic nutrition is important. We need foods from each of the five basic food groups. Make plant foods, such as cereal, grains, vegetables and fruit, the cornerstones of your diet. Don't make the mistake of increasing your portions just because you're eating healthy foods. Excess carbohydrates such as breads are also extra calories that will be stored as fat. Eat moderate amounts of low fat foods from the milk and meat groups. Finally, go sparingly on fats, oils, and sweets.

The greater the lean tissue, the more energy or calories automatically burned off.

The number of calories you consume (energy input) needs to be balanced by the calories you burn off, (energy output). Energy output depends on the basal metabolic rate (rate at which the body uses energy to maintain itself during complete rest), activity metabolic rate (rate at which the body uses energy during activity), and body composition (percentage of lean to percentage of fat tissue). Lean tissue is active tissue and active tissue burns calories. Therefore, the greater the percentage of lean tissue, the more energy or calories automatically burned off. Body fat uses very little energy. Weight training and aerobic exercise not only increase your activity metabolic rate, but also result in a higher basal metabolic rate long after your exercise is complete. In simple terms, you not only benefit during your exercise but long after your exercise is over.

Make good choices. Choose stairs over an elevator. Walk or cycle to the store instead of driving. Park your car some distance from the shopping mall entrance. Spend time with your family during evenings or weekends. Keep on the move and try new things.

FIT & FAT

ENERGY SYSTEMS

Your body has three energy systems that work together to supply it with the energy it needs.

One system is used for very short-lasting activities. An example is getting up from the couch and walking across the room to switch the station on the radio. Your body gets its fuel for this action from carbohydrate sugar stores in your leg muscles.

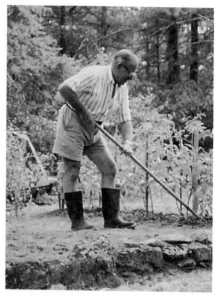

Your body uses its second energy system when you do slightly longer activities that last three to four minutes. Instead of going to the radio, you walk to the kitchen and tidy some dishes. During this activity your body gets its fuel from your blood as well as your muscles.

Once you begin to exercise or work hard, your body turns to a third energy system for help. This is called your aerobic system. This system requires lots of fuel and the more aerobically fit you are, the more fat you use as a fuel source instead of carbohydrates.

When your body is aerobically active you're not only burning fat, you're exercising your heart. These activities are called aerobic exercises and include: walking, swimming, rowing, biking and jogging. You can even activate this fuel system by raking leaves or cleaning your house – providing you are working continuously and at a steady pace.

"An average adult will burn 250-300 calories during one hour of gardening."

MICHELLE LAFRENIERE, YMCA

WHY WE NEED TO EXERCISE:

1. BODY COMPOSITION

Body composition refers to the percentage of body fat compared to lean tissue. Percentage of body fat increases with normal aging. This increase is caused by changes in our bodies' basal metabolic rate and reduced physical activity. Our bodies adapt to specific physical demands placed on them. If we exercise, our bodies meet the demand. And, if we exercise regularly, this results in good long-term effects and our bodies become leaner.

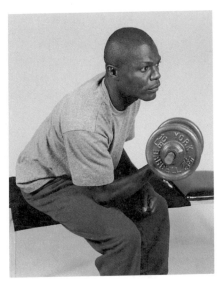

We need to exercise because our body is like a well engineered machine that performs best when it is well serviced and maintained.

2. MUSCLE

Muscle mass naturally starts to decline as early as age 30. It is believed that after age 40, most women lose nearly one quarter of a kilogram (half a pound) of muscle each year. Research proves that strengthening exercises reverse this decline.

3. FLEXIBILITY

Tissues connecting bones together at our joints become stiffer as we age. This reduced flexibility is linked to reduced activity and can also be improved through exercise with a stretching program.

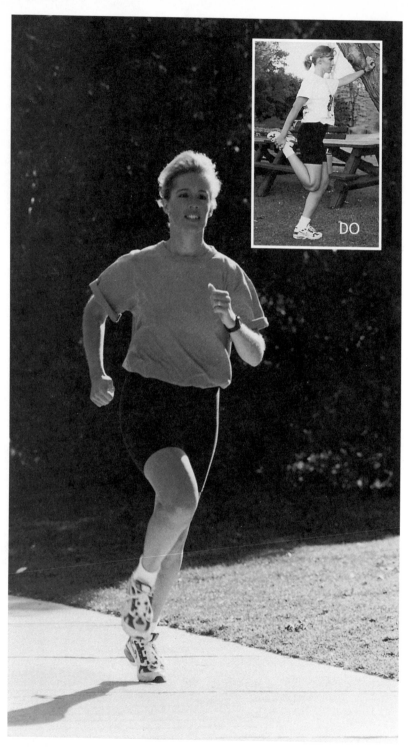

DO

4. BONES

Osteoporosis (thinning bones) concerns everyone. Bones become thinner as we age. Weight bearing exercises such as walking, jogging, and resistive exercises (weight training) are proven to help maintain bone thickness or density. A proper diet and a regular exercise program needs to be introduced early in life to help prevent such problems.

Exercise regularly to keep a lean body, maintain muscle mass, flexibility, strong bones and a healthy heart and lungs.

5. HEART RATE

Your heart is also a muscle and needs to be worked. Our maximum heart rate declines with age. The amount of blood pumped out of the heart per beat increases with exercise and overcomes the effect of a lowered maximum heart rate.

6. OXYGEN UPTAKE

Maximum oxygen uptake (bringing in and using oxygen) declines after the age of 30. Our body's ability to bring in and use oxygen improves with exercise training at any age, and is especially important as we get older. The harder you work these systems, the better and the longer these systems work for you.

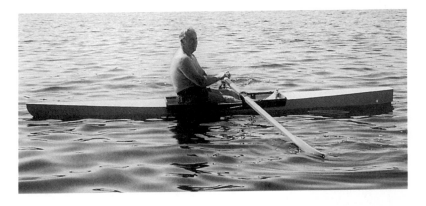

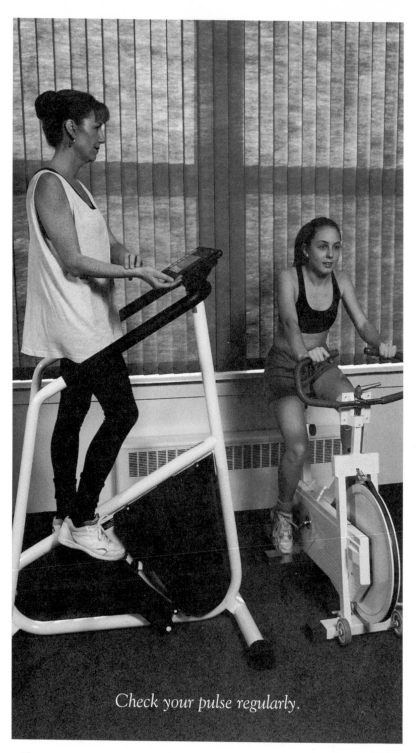

Check your pulse regularly.

AEROBIC EXERCISES

AEROBIC EXERCISES INVOLVE WHOLE BODY ACTIVITY

You use all of your large muscle groups when you walk, jog, or swim. Aerobic exercises are those that safely and comfortably increase your breathing and heart rates for an extended period of time without disturbing the balance between your intake and use of oxygen. Huffing and puffing after you exercise means this balance has been disturbed and you are paying back an oxygen debt. When you perform aerobic exercises correctly you are helping to improve this oxygen delivery system. These steps should be followed when doing aerobic exercises:

Exercise is the recurring theme behind prevention of many key diseases such as heart disease, stroke, diabetes and osteoporosis.

1. RESTING HEART RATE

One of the first signs of improved aerobic fitness is a lower resting heart rate or pulse. Be sure to check your pulse regularly and monitor your improvement over time.

2. WARM-UP

A warm-up lasting three to five minutes prepares your body and muscles for your aerobic workout. Mimicking your chosen activity at an easy pace is a good way to warm up. This will increase the circulation to the muscles that you will soon be using more intensely. Remember also to warm up your muscles before stretching or strengthening exercises. These warm-ups could include five minutes of biking, jogging or walking.

3. TECHNIQUE

Perform your exercise at a steady, moderate pace. Pay attention to your posture and specific details related to your chosen activity. Use good technique.

4. INTENSITY

Studies suggest it is good to exercise within an "aerobic training zone." This means you work just hard enough to have your heart rate enter into your "Target Heart Rate Zone." If you work too hard, the ability of your heart and lungs to supply oxygen to your muscles becomes limited, for they can't keep up with the oxygen demand. There are formulas available to help establish target heart rate zones for adults. Exercise facilities usually post charts illustrating recommended training zones for various age groups. However, there are none so far for children.

5. MONITORING YOUR HEART RATE

You should monitor your heart rate to ensure you remain within your target training zone and to evaluate how long it takes your heart rate to recover after you cool down. Check your pulse just after your warm-up, twice during the aerobic component of your workout and then after cool down. In time, you will recognize the feeling of working within your training zone. The talk test is always a good check to use. As you exercise, you should be able to carry on a normal conversation without sounding out of breath.

6. DURATION AND FREQUENCY

The Institute for Aerobics Research recommends exercising for twenty minutes four times a week, or for thirty minutes three times a week.

Healthy Play Hints

- Establish proper exercise habits and techniques

- Make exercise fun and interesting for young children

- Support your child's interest in organized sports

- Young children should watch less television

- Outdoor play generally improves physical strength

- Encourage your children to participate in activities that use their large muscle groups and last for at least twenty minutes

- Gradually increase the intensity of their exercise

- Encourage aerobic exercise three times a week

- Vary their activities to maintain their interests

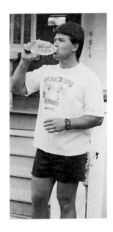

Drink water prior to, during and after exercise.

7. COOL DOWN

Never suddenly stop exercising. Your cool down should take about five minutes and you should slow your exercise to a gradual stop. Your body needs to gradually return to its pre-exercise state.

8. FLUIDS

Drinking extra fluids (hydration) is important when you exercise. Thirst is not a reliable signal. The best drink is water and you should drink prior to, during and after exercise. Hydration is often overlooked by many, young and old. A water bottle is a good gift for your children at Christmas or on birthdays.

AEROBICS FOR CHILDREN

Within the last twelve years, research has focused on the effects of exercise training in children. Children respond to training much the same way as adults do. It is important to get your children interested in exercise and sports early in life. And, the more you get involved, the more likely your children will participate.

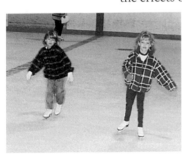

Growing up with an active lifestyle makes a world of difference!

Endurance training is a challenge in the six- to ten-year age group. This younger group does well with activities such as biking, skating, swimming, soccer or a good game of follow the leader.

From age 11 or 12, children are usually mature enough to fully participate and gain full benefit from endurance training. In mid-adolescence, around 16, the greater concern is the teen's loss of interest in physical activity or exercise. Growing up with an active lifestyle can lead to longer-lasting, better habits and make a world of difference!

EXERCISE

For the most part, children and young teenagers do not need a formal exercise program. Regular play and well planned activities allow children to develop normal muscle strength, endurance, co-ordination and balance. Many adults prefer a more formalized or structured exercise routine that will fit into their busy schedules.

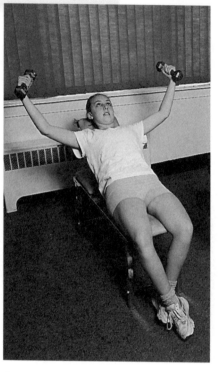

Family activities may include hiking, biking, theme walks (nature, beach, neighbourhood), destination walks/jogs (museum, playground), swimming, and skating. Organized sports also provide young people with many opportunities.

Injuries are an exception and a young person who is injured may require specific strengthening and flexibility exercises. These exercises should be prescribed and monitored by an appropriate health professional.

Some youth-oriented health and fitness facilities offer special programs for young teenagers. Programs include theory and hands-on application of exercise such as strength training, flexibility, and cardiovascular exercises (aerobics). Exercise equipment commonly used by adults is not designed for children. Free weights such as barbells are often the first stage for youth. Strength training with barbells requires responsibility and maturity, as does any formal exercise. Injuries can occur if a person is over-zealous and works with too much weight or increases the weight too quickly. When buying barbells for an enthusiastic teenager, ensure you teach him/her safe and proper use. And finally, most children experience growth spurts between 11 and 15, so make sure your child eats properly to provide the energy needed for his or her level of activity.

EXERCISE

More formalized exercise programs and workouts usually begin during late teens, early twenties and should then become a life-time habit. Exercise is the recurring theme behind prevention of many key diseases such as heart disease, stroke, diabetes and osteoporosis. All of us, at any age, benefit from exercise.

A recent Norwegian medical study found the incidence of breast cancer in women was significantly reduced by regular exercise.

Healthy Play Hints

- Plan backyard play areas to allow for your children's physical play and fitness

- Encourage physical play and participate with your children

- Support your children in organized sports

- Set a good example. Don't be a couch potato!

- Make family fitness activities a regular weekend event – then have a picnic

- Plan birthday parties or extended family gatherings around a special activity such as skating or swimming

- Monitor heavy exercise in 11 to 15 year olds, for their nutritional and water intake must meet their energy requirements

- Remind your children always to warm up and cool down

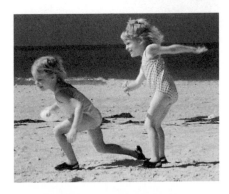

"Those who don't find time for exercise will have to find time for illness."

EARL OF DERBY,
LIVERPOOL, ENGLAND

SPORTS

Don't forget to warm up and cool down for sports, just as you would for any other exercise. Also, it is wise to become familiar with good form and technique specific to the sport you choose. Poor technique and improper warm-ups can result in injuries.

YOUNG ATHLETE

More and more children are involved with competitive sports and as a result, the number of overuse (repetitive action) injuries is increasing. The important difference between the child and adult athlete is that the child is still growing. The bones of their legs, arms and spine grow in length, and the soft tissue, such as muscle and tendon, become longer in response to this bone growth. This results in tightening of the soft tissues. This tightness is most obvious during growth spurts and this is when injuries often occur.

Don't forget to warm up.

Girls usually experience their biggest adolescent growth spurt between 11 and 13 and boys between 13 and 15. The muscle/tendon tightness that accompanies growth spurts makes some children more susceptible to injuries from repetitive stresses such as running. However studies show approximately fifty percent of these injuries are preventable.

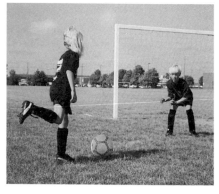

Begin training one to two months prior to your sport's season.

PREVENTION

Begin training one to two months prior to your sport's season beginning. Do not allow more than a ten percent weekly increase in the amount of training time, amount of distance covered or number of repetitions. General fitness exercises must also be part of your training.

The repetitive demands of an activity can lead to muscle imbalances. For example, a distance runner will have tight and strong front thigh muscles (quadriceps) and calf muscles but tight, *weak* muscles at the back of their thighs (hamstrings). If your child is going through a growth spurt, have him or her reduce his or her training load and focus on stretching.

It is important to stretch your hamstring muscles during childhood, adolescence and as an adult. Without stretching, these muscles shorten and may contribute to back problems. Two methods of stretching of hamstrings are shown in the two photos below.

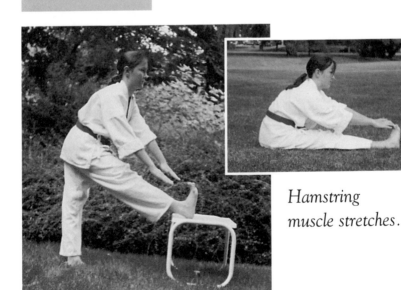

Hamstring muscle stretches.

CHECKLISTS FOR SCHOOL, WORKPLACE & GYM

THE CLASSROOM OR WORKPLACE

Adults spend a great deal of time at work, and our young people spend a great deal of time in school. These checklists have been compiled as an easy reference for all of us. The goal is to learn and practise healthy habits that will last a lifetime.

- Maintain the inward curve in your lower back when sitting

- Interrupt long periods of sitting. Do five back bends every sixty minutes

- Interrupt long periods of deskwork. Do five chin tucks every sixty minutes

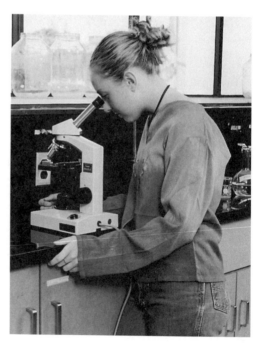

- Interrupt standing bent forward. Do five back bends every thirty minutes

- Interrupt typing. Stretch your fingers, wrists, and shoulders every sixty minutes

- Carry your backpack over both shoulders and walk upright. If heavy, use chest and waist or hip straps

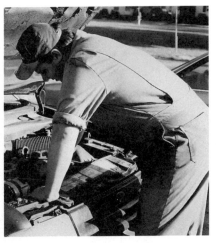

· Keep your elbow slightly bent when carrying a bag

· Stand tall when standing for long periods, and occasionally shift your weight from one foot to the other

· When lifting, bend your knees, keep your back straight, hold object close and do not twist your body

AT THE GYM

· Drink plenty of water

· Always warm up and cool down

· Use safe and effective equipment

· Practise good form and technique

· Do ten 'sloppy' push-ups before and after each abdominal workout

· Do five back bends after all strenuous workouts

· Do five chin tucks when you feel a minor strain in your neck

· When lifting, bend your knees, keep your back straight, hold the weight close and do not twist your body

FINAL CHECKLIST

This final checklist summarizes the key messages found throughout **Body Basics** *for life*. Many are specific and instructional, others are lifestyle suggestions.

· Start and end your day with five 'sloppy' push-ups and five chin tucks

· Sit with an inward curve in your lower back

· Be active everyday

· Drink water before, during, and after physical activity

· Warm up, cool down, and use good technique every time you exercise

· Play hard for thirty minutes three times a week or twenty minutes four times a week

· Always exercise prior to eating

· Do five back bends after all strenuous workouts

· Do ten 'sloppy' push-ups before and after each abdominal workout

· Walking, jogging and weight training strengthens bones

· Eat healthy foods. Limit fatty foods and sweets

· When standing for long periods, stand tall and occasionally shift your weight from one foot to the other

· When lifting, bend your knees, keep your back straight, hold the object close and do not twist your body

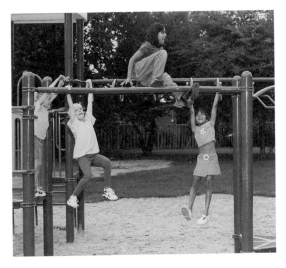

- Carry your backpack over both shoulders, walk upright and use a waist or chest strap if it is heavy

- Keep your elbow slightly bent when carrying a bag

- Interrupt long periods of sitting. Do five back bends every sixty minutes

- Interrupt long periods of desk work. Do five chin tucks every sixty minutes

- Take stretch breaks every sixty minutes when doing repetitive activities

- Be good to your eyes, look up and focus further away every now and then or if you feel eye strain

- When working at a computer, remember to:
    - maintain the inward curve of your back and hold your head upright
    - keep arms at your side, elbows at 90° and your forearms and wrists parallel to the floor
    - sit with the monitor an arm's length away

- Use only one pillow to sleep

MY CLOSING

As I look back through **Body Basics** *for life*, all sorts of thoughts and images come to mind. I picture a lot of neck, back, wrist and shoulder problems caused by prolonged sitting and use of computers, being avoided through easy, proper care of the body. This, of course, is most important for our young people, who are tempted to hunch over electronic games from an early age. It is particularly for them that I have written **Body Basics** *for life*.

On a personal note, my own physical pain forced me to make time for myself. I now exercise regularly and, as a result, have more energy and have conquered my long-standing neck and back pain. I hope this book will help others who suffer, but, more important, will help many more avoid pain altogether. My eight-year-old twin daughters are active, they enjoy sports and both are demonstrating some solid, basic lifestyle habits. At 44, I look forward to a healthy and active life and see the same for them. I'm lucky to have two daughters and a husband who kick-start me to be active — we should all find someone in our life to encourage us to stay active. I am not slowing down, I am just getting started.

You do not need fancy exercise clothes or expensive equipment to feel better. Sitting with good posture and taking a few minutes each day to stretch is a

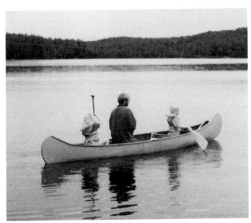

great start. Our body is like a well engineered machine that performs best when it is well serviced and maintained. We all have only one body, so let's do our best to make it last!

Karen Webb

BIBLIOGRAPHY

BOOKS

1. Amen, Karen, *The Crunch*, London, Vermillion, 1994.

2. Bell, Lorna; Seyfer, Eudora, *Gentle Yoga*, Celestial Arts, Berkley, California, 1987.

3. Chalmers Mill, Wendy, *Repetitive Strain Injury*, London, Thorsons, 1994.

4. Cooper, Robert K., *Health & Fitness Excellence: The Scientific Action Plan*, Boston, Houghton Mifflin, 1989.

5. Isernhagen, Susan, *Work Injury Management and Prevention*, Aspen Publishers Inc., Rockland, Maryland 1988.

6. McIlwain, Harris, *Osteoporosis, Prevention Management, Treatment*, New York, Toronto: Wiley, 1988.

7. McKenzie, Robin, *Treat Your Own Back*, Spinal Publications Ltd., New Zealand, 1985.

8. McKenzie, Robin, *Treat Your Own Neck*, Spinal Publications Ltd., New Zealand, 1983.

9. Micelotta, Jeanette, *Get Rid of Your Gut*, New York, Hearst Books, 1993.

10. Nelson, Miriam, Ph.D., *Strong Women Stay Young*, New York, Toronto, Bantam Books, 1997.

11. Roberts, Scott, *Fitness Walking*, Indianapolis, Masters Press, 1995.

12. Vitale, Frank, *Individualized Fitness Programs*, Prentice-Hall Inc., Englewood Cliffs, New Jersey, 1973.

JOURNALS

1. Back Association of Canada, '*Back to Back*', Volume 14, Number 1, March 1994; Volume 14, Number 3, September 1994; Volume 15, Number 2, June 1995; Volume 14, Number 2, June 1994.

2. Brady, Jane, '*Study Links Vigorous Exercise to Longevity*', Globe and Mail, April 19, 1995, New York Times Service.

3. Canadian Press, '*Kids' Fat Intake Linked to TV: Study*', Beacon Herald, Stratford, Ontario, Canada, November 19, 1996.

4. Darden, Ellington Dr., '*Frequently Asked Questions About Muscle, Fat and Exercise*', Athletic Journal 56:20, 85-89, November, 1995.

5. Haywood, Heather Boyce, William, '*Knee Overuse Injuries In The Skeletally Immature Athlete*', Physiotherapy Canada, Summer 1996, Volume 48, Number 3, 190-202.

6. Osteoporosis Society of Canada, '*Physical Activity Fact Sheet Series*', Number 2.

THE PERFECT GIFT THAT SHOWS YOU CARE!

Body Basics *for life, Simple steps to a healthy, pain-free you!* makes a great gift for a friend or for an entire family. A book filled with practical information for everyone, it's great at Christmas, for birthdays, baby showers, graduations, Mother's Day, Father's Day, or any day of the year! Check your local bookstore or order directly from us.

MORE INFORMATION

Educational kits including a book, overhead transparencies and posters are ideal for teaching (primary and secondary schools). These kits will be available during 1998. An information pamphlet for students and their families will also be included. Pamphlets can be photocopied by the school and distributed. We feel parental awareness and support is critical. Please call Birchcliff Publishing Inc. for further details.

MAIL ORDERS

THE PERFECT GIFT THAT SHOWS YOU CARE!

For orders of 5 to 10 books, we'll pay the shipping costs to one address. Just fill out the order form below:

Name
_____

Address
_____

City   Province/State
_____

Postal/Zip Code   Phone
_____

Please send me ____ copies of **Body Basics** *for life* @ $9.95 each	$
Postage & handling $1 per book Orders of 5 to 10 books= No Charge	$
SUBTOTAL	$
Add 7% GST (70¢ per book) Canadian Residents	$
TOTAL AMOUNT ENCLOSED	$

Please make cheque or money order payable to Birchcliff Publishing Inc.

An aggressive discount schedule is available for large volume orders.

- -

GIFT GIVING MADE EASY!

We will send a personally autographed **Body Basics** *for life* directly to the recipient of your choice. Enclose a personal note or card and we will include it with your order.

Please send **Body Basics** *for life* to:

Name
_____

Address
_____

City   Province/State
_____

Postal/Zip Code
_____

MAIL this form along with your payment to:

BIRCHCLIFF PUBLISHING INC.
Suite 126
59 Albert Street
Stratford,
Ontario Canada
N5A 3K2

For more information
CALL:
(519) 273-3334 or
1-888-472-9121 or

FAX:
(519) 273-7222